HOLD FAST TO HOPE

HOLD FAST TO HOPE

Help for Caregivers of Those with Traumatic Injuries

Linda Perrone Rooney, D.Min.

Resurrection Press
An Imprint of
CATHOLIC BOOK PUBLISHING CORP.
Totowa • New Jersey

First Published in March, 2006 by
Catholic Book Publishing/Resurrection Press
77 West End Road
Totowa, NJ 07512

ISBN 1-933066-03-2

Library of Congress Catalog Card Number: 2006920925

Cover design by Beth DeNapoli

Printed in the United States of America

1 2 3 4 5 6 7 8 9

www.catholicbookpublishing.com

DEDICATION

To Joe, my inspiration and dear love whose whole life was a story of faith lived with grace and joy, and to all those whose courageous faith and unquenchable hope witness to God's loving presence, even in the midst of intolerable suffering.

ACKNOWLEDGMENTS

I want to thank all those whose encouragement and support over the years enabled me to write this book. Chief among them is my husband, Joe Rooney, who died earlier this year. His unswerving enthusiasm in support of my dreams throughout our marriage was a gift that continues to give, even now.

As well, I thank my family and friends, especially my mother, Gertrude Perrone, and Rochelle Bennett, who never failed to tell me this was an important and needed topic. My editor, Emilie Cerar, is the kind of editor one hopes to have . . . steadying shaky nerves, guiding editorial decisions and encouraging each step of the way.

Contents

Foreword

MOST of us avoid thinking about death or dying. When we do allow our thoughts to turn to the reality of the end of life, we tend to view its arrival on our terms after a long, fruitful life and after all our affairs are in order. A traumatic injury immediately changes this view. When we, or someone we love experiences trauma, everything is turned upside down. Dreams and plans are shattered. The new order for the day is unraveling the mysteries of high-tech medical care and finding ways to pay for it. For anyone living through the turmoil of such an experience, Linda Rooney offers practical ways to sustain hope and survive.

Because of her personal experience following her husband's accident and subsequent brain injury, and her training as a Catholic chaplain, Linda displays a keen appreciation of the needs of the family members of those who suffer from traumatic brain injury. While hospital personnel work frantically to save the life of the person injured, family members must deal with the emotional, physical and financial aspects of what has happened, as well as the pressures of straddling the world of medical institutions and the everyday world of family and work. Linda addresses this tension. She explains what it is like to hear a group of doctors discuss her husband's condition and then tell her in cold, clinical terms what his chances for survival are. To medical personnel he is a patient and there is little recognition of the familial bonds that tie him to a larger world, a world of intimacy and love. Linda is the one who must keep her husband's story alive.

This is a book filled with practical advice on how to keep hope alive, not only for the patient in the hospital, but also for the patient's family by attending to, rather than ignoring the many small details of living. Linda reminds caregivers that hope means appreciating God's presence wherever one finds it. She gives step-by-step advice on how to cope, such as allowing others to help, asking to see your loved one, and keeping your thoughts positive. Whether it is dealing with one's feelings or asserting oneself with medical personnel, Linda encourages the caregiver to be proactive.

The two pillars that support this book's approach to hope are "facts" and "prayer." Hope is not built on an illusion but on a correct understanding of reality. Linda provides facts about brain injury as well as a list of resources where one can go for more information. She also empowers patients and family members by informing them about their bill of rights and encourages them to actively participate in health-care decision-making. But she recognizes that there is much more to us as human persons than what the medical community can offer. We also have a spiritual dimension that needs to be nourished by prayer and she provides us with prayers and rituals to assist us on the journey.

One can't help but think of church as a community of the faithful when reading this book. Here we find a member of the community who has undergone tremendous suffering and hardship, but rather than dwell on her personal loss, she turns her grief away from herself and uses it in the service of others. In the process, she, herself, becomes a source of hope.

—Marilyn Martone, Ph.D.

Prologue

ON June 28, 1997, my husband, Joe, on the return lap of a two-hour bike ride around Winona, Minnesota, suffered a cardiac arrest that threw him to the ground, smashing his skull. Bystanders said he "fell like a rock." He was not wearing a helmet and suffered massive damage to the right temporal lobe of his brain. For all intents and purposes, he was dead when he hit the ground; he was not breathing, nor did he have a pulse. A person in the crowd rushed to his side and applied CPR, keeping him alive until the paramedics arrived. They administered a defibrillator twice on the way to the local emergency room and because of their competent efforts he stabilized and was delivered by helicopter to the Mayo Clinic, in nearby Rochester, Minnesota.

While this life-changing event was occurring, I was preparing to teach a graduate course at St. Mary's University. Ironically, though he normally wore a helmet, Joe failed to rent one that day and promised to do so after his ride was finished. With this agreement tucked away in my heart, I kissed him and watched him ride off to enjoy the lovely summer day. I can still see his strong back peddling down the hill with athletic grace and confidence. It's the last I saw of the man I married. The man who survived this tragic event, while having made miraculous progress, became a different man.

This book is born of the pain and joy of my own experience. It is a collection of reflections, prayers and practical advice that I hope will bring comfort, strength and healing to families who struggle to care for a loved one who has suffered a traumatic injury and is in some stage of rehabilitation.

I've chosen to write this book for several reasons. First, I am a nationally certified Catholic chaplain and because of that I am aware of and want to share resources that should and can be available to families keeping vigil. I also have the personal experience of surviving this catastrophic event and I've learned some important lessons about self-care that are often forgotten in the intensity of caring for another. Finally, I believe we need to create a circle of care around caregivers who are often forgotten sufferers in situations where so much attention is given to the one who is ill.

You can approach this book in a number of ways.

- Read it cover to cover, allowing those things that find a place in your heart to dwell there and add to your healing.
- Scan the table of contents and begin with a chapter that calls to you. In this way, you use the reflections to meet your daily needs and feelings.
- Flip through the book until a particular prayer, subtitle or chapter heading captures your attention.

In other words, there is no correct way to use this book. If all you do is hold it on your lap as a reminder that someone else has walked this path before you, and survived, it will have served its purpose.

I hope those in the medical profession who read this book grow in their ability to understand and extend empathy to patients and their families, just as they extend medical competence. I pray that they will see that the healing needed by the human person involves not only the body and the mind, but also, the spirit. The very best medical caregivers for my husband were those who also cared for me and allowed me not only to be a member of the therapeutic team; but also, a person in need of kindness, honesty and at least a modicum of participation in my husband's medical decisions. The very best medical personnel were not only competent; they were compassionate, collaborative and able to communicate at all levels.

Be assured that as you read these words I am praying for all those critically ill, their medical and spiritual caregivers and families. Open yourself to those prayers and allow the power of God's Spirit to carry you on.

A Prayer Before Reading

Gentle and Loving God, so much has happened in our lives. I am overwhelmed by events over which I have no control. I know you hold us in the palm of your hand, and I want to rest there. There are so many changes and stresses that pull me away from you and away from the inner peace you want me to have. Give me a calm spirit as I read this book. Allow me to hear what I need most. Show me where I need to grow. Give me strength to do what I will learn I must do.

Comfort me in the deepest places of my fear and hurt. Be with me today as you have been with me each day of my life. Heal my loved one. Grant me a willing spirit ready to embrace your will. Amen.

Chapter 1

A God of Life and Healing

In her book, *Finding Our Way Home,* K. Killian Noe observes that:

> *In order for someone to make the shift into a radically new way of life, he or she has to really want a new way of life. There has to have been a moment of decision, of choosing for oneself. It can't be something chosen under pressure or chosen for one's mother or father or husband or best friend. It has to be a choosing that comes from one's own depths. When Jesus approached the man at the sheep gate pool who had been crippled for thirty-eight years, the first question Jesus asked him was, 'Do you want to be healed? Do you want to be free?' You'd think the answer to the question would be an obvious yes, but that's not necessarily so.*

CAREGIVERS do not choose their role. They do not sort among their many options, for the options of the caregivers of those with traumatic injuries are few. Caregivers are drafted into their role by the nature of their relationships. It takes every minute of every day for many months and years. For some, it takes a lifetime.

Yet, caregivers do have choices. They can be healed in the midst of being healers. Their choices center on what kind of person they want to be, how they want to honor their relationship with the one injured, what inner resources they have that have not been fully plumbed, and to what degree they want their values to shape the harsh reality of life.

The God of most major religions is one who cares—who brought into being all of creation and sustains it in life until it is time, within its natural cycle, to die.

As a Catholic Christian, I believe in a God of life and healing. I believe that the God who gave me life also gives me everything I need to live that life successfully. I believe that I was given the gift of making free choices and that each choice I make either reinforces good and sustains the quality of life; or weakens good and detracts from that quality, not only for me, but also for all those whom my decisions affect. Either way, I make the choices.

In the midst of the overwhelming fatigue and challenges of caring for another, faith plays a pivotal role in determining whether or not the caregiver can give what is needed over the long haul. The kind of God we believe in helps or hinders that process.

How Do We Recognize God in the Midst of Suffering?

Even for those who profess a belief in God, recognizing God's presence in the midst of suffering is a difficult task. First we look for a miracle—something or someone who will take all of this misery away. Then, after we come to grips with the fact that this traumatic event is not a dream and will not go away, we simply look for strength and comfort. We may experience anger at God for allowing such events to happen. We may toss our faith away for a time, thinking we have believed in vain. Many people cling to faith. They saturate themselves with as much prayer and spiritual nourishment as they can access. They ask family and friends and even total strangers to pray for their loved one and themselves. They visit the hospital chapel, request the presence of a chaplain, fill the room with artifacts and objects of their faith in the hope that a strong show of faith will deter God's wrath and bring God's blessing. For some, this is bargaining. For others, they are genuine gestures of faith in God's mercy and healing.

The fact is that God's presence doesn't often come in miraculous apparitions or cures. Few will see God face to face or hear the magic words that make everything better. Rather, God's presence comes in quiet moments, through the presence of others who care and through the use of spiritual resources such as books on prayer, scripture and healing. A look at each of these gives us clues that can assist us in finding God's presence when we are engulfed in suffering, anxiety and confusion.

Quiet

Americans are surrounded by noise, frenetic activity and multiple and simultaneous demands. We pride ourselves on being able to multitask, that is, do more than one thing at the same time. Imagine for a minute the average working parent who hustles kids into a car while finishing a business call on the phone, and signing off on homework. It's a typical scene in millions of homes daily. For some reason, we have accepted the value of multitasking without thinking about its consequences.

One of its consequences is a decrease or absolute lack of quiet in our lives. Worse, many have become uncomfortable with silence, with times of quiet, with solitude. This discomfort plays a key role in our inability to experience the presence of God, to hear his voice and to recognize His direction.

In the midst of caring for another, we might intellectually yearn for quiet and solitude; yet we seldom build it into our day. Why is that? Perhaps we are afraid to meet God and to hear his words of consolation. Perhaps the struggle to care seems jeopardized if our own comfort is sought. Perhaps we fear we will not receive comfort, but some awful reprimand. Whatever it is that holds us back from taking time for quiet and solitude in the midst of our caregiving, to do so defeats our desire to experience God's mercy and consolation.

When we take time to sit quietly, to breathe deeply and to become attuned to the sacredness of the space in which we reside, God's spirit of peace, strength and compassion has the opportunity to break through the chaos and rest gently within us. The habit of seeking God's solace builds in us a reservoir from which we can draw wisdom and courage for the day ahead.

The Presence of Others Who Care

It should be no surprise that we can and will experience God through others. Our God became a human being, in Jesus Christ, for that very reason, so that we could experience God through our human senses and come to be strengthened in faith.

There are many whose presence is God's gift to us. Medical personnel who care for the spirit as well as the body, family and friends who stay in touch and help us with myriad details, church members who send encouragement and prayers, neighbors who bring meals and empathy, co-workers who free our time by assuming some of our work, employers who help us to develop flexible work hours, and hundreds of others whose gestures, words, and kindness form a cocoon in which we can be healed as we heal others. All are images of God's presence reaching out to us.

Spiritual Resources

In every religion there are books, prayers, devotionals and symbols that offer healing and peace. Pick up a book and allow someone else to assist you in understanding the work of the spirit during difficult times. Recite prayers, even if your heart is heavy and in doubt. As you listen to the words and offer the heartfelt gesture, you will be blest by the experience that others know how you feel and have put those feelings into words you cannot yet express. Use whatever symbols or devotionals are important to your faith system, for they come from years of tradition that have proven effective in aiding the soul to communicate with God.

Catholicism is rich in spiritual resources. The Bible, meditation and prayer books, the Liturgy of the Hours, Mass, the rosary, the Stations of the Cross, the sacraments, especially the Sacrament of the Sick are all avenues to God's presence. Using them prepares the heart, soul and mind to receive inspiration. Start with the prayers and rituals at the end of this book. If you are unaccustomed to prayer in your life, begin slowly. God invites you into deep conversation and longs to wrap you in love. Your effort to be open to God's presence will be rewarded.

Whom Do You Seek?

In the Hebrew Scriptures, many seekers encountered God. Abraham's son was spared death because Abraham met God in three strangers and followed their command. Noah's family survived the great flood because they listened to God's guidance. Moses met God in a burning bush, listened to God's voice and followed the commandments. The great prophets, even though they were often afraid and felt ill-equipped for the task, took courage in God's presence and became God's messengers.

In the Christian Scriptures, God took this loving presence one step further, and sent God's Son, Jesus Christ, to show this divine love and mercy in the flesh. The Jews were looking for a military messiah who would save Israel from the Romans. They missed God's presence in the carpenter whose words and actions seemed unbelievable.

Yet, some believed. Mary and Joseph placed their lives in God's hands and were rewarded with the love of their son, Jesus. Peter, John, Mary Magdalene and the others who followed Jesus changed their lives in order to become a person worthy of God's presence in Christ. After his death, a religion formed that gave its members the courage to face wild beasts and to endure persecution and suffering with joy.

Surely, if God has found ways throughout all of history to make this divine presence known, then we who seek, will find God in the suffering we witness each day in the body and spirit of our loved one and in the midst of our own emotional, physical and spiritual ennui.

God of joy and sadness, be with me. Hold my heart in your comforting embrace for it is breaking from sorrow, fear and the weight of all that is happening in our lives. I need to believe in your healing power and in your sustaining presence. Fill me with hope and strengthen my faith. Amen.

Take a few minutes to reflect on and describe the God in whom you believe. Is God one who loves and comforts you, one who is with you always, especially during difficult times? Do you believe that God is a God of hope and healing? During this time, write your own prayers using the feelings of your heart and the words of your faith.

Chapter Two

Tell Your Story: Let Healing Begin

The first step to healing is telling your story. You need to trace and remember the details of your experience so that you can share them with your loved one later. The telling and retelling helps you to identify your feelings and to sort out the sequence of events and decisions. Eventually, when your loved one is able, you can share those first hours, since it is likely that he/she won't remember what happened. Try to remember both the factual details and the emotions involved. If you can, keep a journal and take pictures.

Linda's Story

ON the day Joe suffered his brain injury, I was in the student center of St. Mary's University, Winona, Minnesota, using the computer to complete a handout for my class that would meet one hour later. As I worked, the student receptionist answered the phone and I heard her say, "Yes, she teaches here. Just a minute while I check on her room number (pause). She's staying in the apartments, #7, but I'm not sure if she's there now." As she mentioned the apartment number I realized she was talking about me. I indicated, quietly, that I was Dr. Rooney. She kept listening on the phone while holding up her finger for me to wait. Shortly, she hung up the phone. "Are you Dr. Rooney?" she asked. "Yes," I said, "was that call for me?" "Yes it was," she answered. "There is a flower delivery they're trying to make and they want to be sure you're available to receive it. They want you to wait here. Someone is coming right over." "Ok," I said. "I still have some computer work to do so I'll be right here."

I returned to my workstation and began to type. As I worked two things flashed through my mind. The first was, "I hope this doesn't have anything to do with Joe." My subconscious was aware that I hadn't seen him in two hours. The other thought was, "who would be sending us flowers up here?" Even though we had celebrated our fifteenth wedding anniversary two days before, I didn't expect anyone to remember it. In that subconscious desire to solve the mystery of the phone call, I was ready to accept any answer that was positive. As a matter of fact, I said a little prayer that the "delivery" would not be bad news. It continues to amaze me that my intuitive self realized that call had nothing to do with flowers.

As I stood near the computer proofreading my work, the outside glass door opened and a police officer entered the building. As soon as I saw him I knew he was looking for me. I felt my heart begin to race and the muscles in my body tighten. The many times I had stood with families in emergency rooms as their chaplain while someone told them bad news, flashed through my mind. I tried to tell myself to stay calm so that I could get the information I needed to deal with whatever had happened. The officer approached the counter asking for Mrs. Rooney and if there was somewhere more private where we could talk. With those words, my life changed forever. I was aware that my body felt weakened, as though I had received a physical blow. Even as I showed him into a nearby empty classroom, I felt as though I was outside my body watching two people I didn't know.

The police officer did his best to tell me the difficult news. He began to describe the situation and had hardly begun when I said, "Please, before you go any further, tell me whether my husband is alive or dead. Knowing this will change how I am able to listen to you." He hesitated and then said, "When they put him on the helicopter he was alive. I'm not sure of the situation after that." Once I had the basic information I thanked him for the caring way in which he delivered it. He asked if I was ok and assured that I was, he left. Throughout that encounter, I was calm, tear-free and in control.

Decision One: Tell someone the news.

When he left the room, I slumped against the desk trying to collect my thoughts and determine what to do next. My brain felt trapped in slow motion. For about 30 seconds I couldn't manage conscious, coordinated thought. Just as this began to scare me, I realized I needed to find the Director of the Graduate Program, ask for help and find a way to travel to the hospital. As I hurried down the hall and turned the corner, I saw him talking with a student. I asked if I could see him for a moment and we moved aside. Up until this time I had been calm. As I began to describe what had happened, I could barely get the words out. All I could say, at first, was, "Something has happened to Joe." I think I repeated it at least three times before I could tell him what happened. As I finished a brief sketch of events, I burst into tears. Finally, the emotion was being released. The tears didn't last long because my mind kept telling me to "get a grip" and figure out a plan of action. From somewhere deep inside I realized I needed to call our sons, and I asked for help to make the calls.

Decision Two: Contact those close to you.

With help from the staff, I approached the phones just as a call came in for me. It was our son, Dan, calling to say they knew what happened and were trying to get plane tickets to fly from Orlando, Florida, to Rochester, Minnesota. I updated him with what I knew and felt bolstered by the fact that I would not be alone to face the next few days. At that moment there was no one else to call. Because my brother was being married that same day, I didn't want to ruin their joy with our sorrow, so I rationalized that extended family could be called when we knew more of what to tell them. As the hours passed, I realized the wisdom of this decision.

Decision Three: Allow others to help.

While I was on the phone, other faculty and friends arrived to offer me their support, prayers and help. The Associate Director of the Program agreed to drive me to the Mayo Clinic, one hour away, and to stay with me as long as necessary. I had known these people for a total of seven days but they would support me as family over the next month. While they made arrangements for the drive, I called the local hospital emergency room and spoke with the doctor who had stabilized Joe. I wrote down what he said because I knew the family would want to know the details. I needed to know, too. Then Michael, our physician son, called and the details I had helped him to communicate better with the emergency room doctor at the Mayo clinic. Between us, we were able to piece together a beginning picture of what I would be facing when I arrived. It was a somber, horrific picture but I consciously didn't let myself dwell on it. All I was aware of was a deep need to hurry to the hospital so that Joe wouldn't be alone.

A staff member volunteered to take my class, and I went to get Joe's bag of medicines, his rosary, prayer book and wallet with his insurance cards. I packed a few days of essentials for myself, a book, notebook and address book and ran back to the car. My driver kept up a stream of dialogue and I found myself responding. It crossed my mind that I was in shock because the situation didn't seem real; I alternated between wanting to cry and wanting to laugh. We broke the speed limit and on route, Michael called again to tell me what was happening in Florida and to give me the latest update from Mayo. The second update was far worse than the first, and I could hear in Michael's voice the tension of not wanting to tell me everything. I didn't ask him to . . . I really didn't want to know.

Decision Four: Determine treatment.

As I identified myself, the nurse said, "I'm so glad you're here, the doctor has been waiting for you." A surgeon arrived and proceeded to tell me in a kind but direct way that Joe was in serious trouble. "Mrs. Rooney, your husband has suffered a massive trauma to the brain. Right now, that is the most life threatening of his injuries. We think he suffered a cardiac arrest but we really can't treat his heart until we've dealt with his brain. I am suggesting that we remove his right temporal lobe, immediately." I remember feeling an inner calm that wanted to say, "go ahead, do anything as long as you save him." What I said, however, was: "Doctor, if you do this operation, what are his chances?" He said, "Right now, I don't know but I would say 50-50 that he will regain a reasonable life." It struck me that he said, "a reasonable life." I asked him, "What do you mean by a reasonable life? Will he be able to function on his own and have any quality to his life?"

My husband and I had talked many times about the quality of life we would want to sustain should anything awful happen to either of us. I wanted to honor his wishes, if necessary. "Doctor, what are my options here?" "Mrs. Rooney, you really don't have any options. If we don't operate on your husband very soon his brain will herniate, crushing his spinal cord and he will die." The bottom line was very clear; yet, I found myself reverting to my chaplain role, mentally reviewing the moral boundaries associated with this kind of case. I knew I did not have to use any extraordinary means to save him if in doing so he would be left in an irreversible vegetative state and/or the burden of the situation would cause grave repercussions for the family.

Everything was buzzing around in my head at once while the doctor waited. I knew what I wanted to do but I wanted someone else's opinion, too. As a stepmother, it seemed only right to have one of the boys bear the decision with me so that in the future it would not be a stumbling block if things did not go well. I called Michael and after we talked he said: "Linda, whatever you decide we will support 100%. This is a very difficult decision. There are no guarantees, but I would go for the operation." That was the same decision I had already made. I reasoned that I owed Joe that 50-50 chance. Having the support lifted the burden and allowed me greater strength to deal with the consequences.

Decision Five: Ask to see your loved one.

Once I told the doctor to proceed with surgery, he rose to leave. I asked if I could see Joe. He hesitated and said that he was in terrible shape and I wouldn't want to see him looking as he did. I replied, "Doctor, this is my husband. I've worked in emergency rooms helping lots of other people claim their loved ones. I can do whatever is necessary now. I don't want him to go to surgery without seeing him. It may be the last time I see him alive." He led me into the cubicle and the form I saw stretched out before me bore no resemblance to my healthy, handsome husband. Had I not known it was Joe and recognized his clothing and wedding ring, I would have been hard pressed to identify him. His clothing, chest area, hands and legs were bloody and scraped from the fall. His head was the size of a basketball, distorting the features beyond recognition. He was, of course, unconscious and inert. We had lost a lot, but we were going to go through this together and that gave me strength.

Decision Six: Keep your thoughts positive and reassuring.

I took Joe's hand and remembering that often patients can hear you even when unconscious, I spoke into his ear. "Joe, it's Linda. I'm here now and I love you. You've had a bad fall from your bike but the doctor is going to do surgery and fix things up. You're hurt pretty bad, Joe, but I know you can make it if you give it your best try. Remember how much we all love you. The Lord loves you, Joe, and He has sent his angels to watch out for you. Don't be afraid, your guardian angel is with you, taking care of you. Your angel, Patrick (a family joke), is going to be with you every step of the way. I'll be here waiting for the surgery to be over and I want to hear good news. I love you very much and I always will." As I stepped back they wheeled him away.

Decision Seven: Take care of details: admissions, insurance and belongings.

I returned to the waiting room where a nurse asked if I wanted to deal with admissions now or wait until later. I chose to get things done before anything else happened. She entered Joe's information onto the computer along with his Medicare and Supplemental Insurance. I gave the nurse his medicines and answered questions about allergies, etc. Back in the waiting room she brought a bag containing Joe's belongings. Seeing his personal effects, his wedding band, watch, biking clothes, shoes, wallet, and the cross I had given him, tore my heart out. Now I sobbed. It was cathartic to cry; everything in me wanted to simply give in to my grief and fear except for some small voice that urged me to just hold on. My mind kept asking, "What will I do without Joe? How will I cope if he cannot recover? What will become of us?" The only answer that emerged was, "I am with you always even to the end of time." It was enough for the moment.

Decision Eight: Endure the long wait.

The next stop was the Neurological Intensive Care Unit where two individual units of 10 glass rooms, in semi-circular configuration around a nursing station, converged. On the other side of a long corridor were private waiting rooms assigned to families for the early stages of their waiting, a lounge with refrigerator, microwave, snacks, TV, magazines and comfortable sleeping chairs, as well as restrooms with showers. It was a self-contained "staging area" where families could try to find some semblance of order, comfort, rest and self-care while they kept 24-hour vigil over their loved one. I only came to appreciate this arrangement several days after Joe's surgery when my own brain began to function more normally, and I actually noticed the world around me. During these first hours, I was unaware of anything but the private waiting room, with its couch, lounge chair, TV and phone, that had our name on the outside of the door. It was from this small womb that I called co-workers and Joe's family. I only had energy for a few calls and I realized two things as I made those calls:

1. Each call drained my emotional reserve and I knew I needed that energy to face the results of the surgery. I needed to prioritize who should be called.
2. With each telling of the details, what was until then a surreal, slow- moving film became an unthinkable reality.

After several hours, our surgeon came to the room and informed me that the surgery had gone as well as possible. Joe had "held his own" and needed no resuscitation efforts. They had removed his right temporal lobe and the future was uncertain. We learned that the next few days would provide a guidepost for what to expect. For now, Joe was alive and in a while I could see him in his intensive care room.

Decision Nine: Get some rest.

My heart sighed at this news. I knew hope. It was fragile and I kept telling myself not to cling to it because it might be short-lived. Yet even my pragmatic alter ego could not rob me of that burst of energy that comes when you have somehow avoided the expected "worse case scenario." Joe was alive. Tomorrow was another day. I prayed in thanksgiving for the miracle that had been granted this day and for all those who had contributed to it. Then I settled down to rest while I waited for the boys to arrive and a new day to begin. It's important to take one day at a time.

God of our fathers and mothers, be with me now. The doctors give information I don't always understand. I am tired but unable to truly rest. There are so many decisions to make. Please give me the wisdom to do the right thing for my loved one. Be with me, O God. Be my light and my salvation. Protect and heal my loved one. Be with us each moment of every day. Amen.

At this time, stop reading and in a notebook or journal, write your own story and the decisions you made.

Chapter Three

Make Friends with Your Feelings

If you are a human being, you have feelings. It's that simple. Along the way some of us received messages that only certain feelings were useful and acceptable. Those messages were wrong. All feelings are important to pay attention to and to claim. When someone you love suffers you experience a multitude of feelings. Denying them or running from them only makes the situation worse. It robs you of the opportunity to claim your experience and to allow it to carve in you a deeper life, a richer character. Whatever happens, be gentle with yourself.

FOR many years I've taught courses on communication skills, assertive communication, pastoral communication, anger and conflict management. One of my favorite lines is: "Feelings are facts. They are neither bad nor good; they just are. What you do with them makes the difference between having them as friends or having them as enemies."

While I've always believed this, I have learned its wisdom through personal as well as professional encounters. It has truly become a "mantra" for me since my husband's accident. Our feelings *can* be our friends; assisting us in our own self-care as well as the care we give to our loved one. They can also be our enemy if we do not take them seriously or refuse to pay attention to our inner emotional life. When we ignore or deny our feelings they have the power to become unconscious behaviors. We can "act out" what is un-named or unresolved within us in ways that both add to our own inner stress and damage relationships with those around us.

Normal Feelings in a Traumatic Situation

When a person experiences a traumatic event, and especially when that trauma involves a loved one hanging between life and death, there are many emotions which are perfectly normal to feel. These include fear, disbelief, sadness, shock, self-pity, anger, numbness, panic, grief, confusion, disorientation, denial, stoicism, withdrawal, anxiety and depression.

I've selected some of these feelings to explore more fully because I believe they are sometimes more difficult for the average person to recognize and to accept. Each person's experience is, of course, unique, so let these thoughts be a beginning point for your own self-reflection and self-understanding.

Shock and Disbelief: *Shock is experienced as numbness, living in a cloud, functioning on remote control without experiencing the feelings that accompany actions or the clear thoughts that precede decisions. Disbelief is an experience of knowing the facts of a situation but not really believing them deep down. We know certain things are true but we repeatedly need to be reminded of that.*

In the first few hours after I was notified about the seriousness of Joe's accident, I functioned in a fog-like zone of unreality. Of course I was aware of what had happened. Of course I knew how close my husband was to death. Yet, it seemed somewhat like an impressionist's rendition of reality: slightly blurred and at close range unrecognizable.

As information floated in and the hours became days I fluctuated between exhaustion and numbness. I spent every possible hour at the hospital, leaving Joe's room only to eat or to go back to my room for the night. The physical toll of little sleep, poor nutrition, no exercise and nothing meaningful to do, compounded by the endless waiting, boredom and anxiety, made my nerves raw. I began to see the edge of irritability rise when nurses were not gentle with him or when they asked me to leave the room for a perfectly good reason. Things that ordinarily would not bother me were suddenly earth-shattering. I could see what I was doing but I didn't seem to have control over my own reactions. I kept expecting to walk into his room and find everything back to normal. It took a while to accept that normal had just changed 360 degrees.

Depression: *Depression is an emotional state characterized by withdrawal from social interaction, repressed anger, inability to communicate one's concerns or feelings.*

As the days became weeks, Joe emerged from his coma and began to move to the first stages of recovery. It became very clear that recovery was a relative thing and that whatever recovery would happen would take a long, long time. As this truth settled in, I began to experience a mild depression. I became aware of it when I suddenly realized that I was only eating one meal each day; I wasn't sleeping more than a few fitful hours each night; and I was withdrawing from contact with family and friends. Part of me needed contact and part of me did not want to talk with anyone. I found myself angry when asked questions about Joe's physical and mental recovery. I wanted to protect him from people's questions and pity. Yet, I knew that many were concerned and deserved information. At the same time, I was angry at Joe because he did not know me. With that came the guilt of blaming someone who was without the cognitive and physical ability to talk let alone choose to not know me. The guilt and shame at having these feelings had nowhere to go but within. I didn't really have someone to talk to that I thought would understand and so the feelings went underground and depression became something I had to really fight against.

If you begin to recognize some of these signs of depression: withdrawal, exhaustion or unusual fatigue, uncontrollable anger, weeping, trouble eating/sleeping, the best thing you can do is to find someone to talk with about what is happening in your life. This may be a trusted friend or family member; or, you may need to seek out a therapist. If they do not approach you first, you may want to seek out the hospital social worker or chaplain. They are usually trained to help identify problems and to work with a person to find coping resources.

Don't try to "go it alone." It is definitely the hard way and doesn't always work.

Anger: *Anger is a normal emotion that is the result of frustration of one's needs or goals, or an attack on one's self-esteem.*

Anger is one of those emotions many people grow up trying not to show, especially if they are women. Women are taught from an early age that anger is not "polite" or "nice" and that girls who show their anger won't be liked by others, especially boys. Boys often get the opposite message. They are taught that their aggressive behavior is the stuff of which men are made. If a man gets angry he is showing his strength. If a woman gets angry she is called nasty names. As a result, many women hide from their anger by becoming passive or by pretending to be calm and non-conflicted all the while holding their anger inside. Often this leads to depressive episodes and/or physical or emotional problems.

I was lucky in several ways when I became aware of my anger. First of all, I came from a family where anger was often on the table and both men and women expressed it. While not all my experiences of anger within my family of origin were healthy, the fact that I saw both men and women express anger and still be accepted gave me a signal that I could express it, too, and not lose my ability to be loved and loveable. Secondly, my dad bolstered my self-confidence and gave me consistent messages that I was a capable person who could and should hold her own with anyone. Self-confidence is a quality that cannot be underestimated in the development of a child. It helps conquer many obstacles in life. Third, I have been educated in the inner dynamics of the human person and in the peculiarities of the emotions, especially anger.

While I could not always predict and control my anger during the early and even later stages of my husband's recovery, I did understand what was happening and gradually was able to control the tumultuous emotional upheaval I was undergoing. Accepting anger as a natural part of human emotional makeup and accepting myself as having both reason to be angry and the ability to choose to use my anger in a positive way, allowed me to overcome the more destructive elements of anger that were not claimed and to make it my friend during the early days of this situation.

Things to understand about anger:

- Anger is neither bad nor good; it simply is.
- Anger is a normal emotion and is morally neutral.
- Anger is the result of frustration, powerlessness, thwarted goals or threatened self-esteem
- Anger can be a powerful friend or a powerful enemy

Fight or Flight

When the psyche comes under stress there are two primary responses it wants to make: fight or flight. Understanding these responses opens up our options and allows us to choose the response that will best help us through difficult situations.

Fight: In this internal response, we make a decision to "stand our ground" and battle for our goals. We might do this mentally by developing an argument; verbally, by arguing and/or yelling at our "opponent;" or even physically, by engaging in aggressive behavior. When we turn loose our anger into a "fight response" everyone loses. We lose because seldom are we taken seriously enough for our truth or feelings to be heard and respected. The other person loses because they, too, are unable to convey their needs in a way that promotes dialogue. In the case of a patient we love, they lose, too, because they cease to remain the focus of the interaction and simply become an appendage to those who are fighting. As caregivers, our responsibility to advocate for our loved one must be the primary focus of the way in which we respond to medical personnel, insurance companies, and anyone else who has the ability to affect their lives. Fighting does not achieve this goal. Often it sets things back or causes the system working for our loved one to break down permanently or long enough to jeopardize their well-being physically, mentally, emotionally or financially.

Flight: This response is demonstrated by physical, mental or emotional withdrawal. Instead of "standing our ground" we run from the situation. It is the passive side of anger. When we are in a state of emotional flight we fail to talk about our feelings and thoughts with concerned others. We may leave the room or find excuses not to visit or spend time with our loved one. We might look for ways to have others care for our loved one rather than be faced with the reality of their condition or recovery. Flight is a damaging response to our anxieties and anger because it internalizes our feelings rather than constructively understanding and dealing with them.

Ways to Make Your Feelings Your Friends

1. **Name them.** When you can name your feelings you are on the road to understanding them and then making sensible choices regarding how you want to act in relation to them. For example: If you are sad, say you are sad; not that you are fine. Those who have difficulty expressing their feelings should take comfort in the knowledge that the uncomfortable feelings that accompany talking about feelings will improve with practice. Most people have a very limited feeling vocabulary. The list at the end of this chapter will help you to expand your feeling vocabulary so that you can more clearly name your feelings to yourself and others.

2. **Claim them.** Once you have named how you feel, allow yourself to accept that feeling without trying to defend or deny it. For example, if you are angry, accept your anger and don't tell yourself you "shouldn't feel that way;" or, "it's a bad thing to feel." Don't deny what you feel because someone else wouldn't approve or agree. Own who you are by claiming what you feel. It is a liberating experience that builds confidence in addition to helping you to act with behaviors consistent with your feelings. It helps others know how to respond to you, too, and enables a more genuine, helpful and honest exchange.

3. **Tame them.** Once named and accepted, feelings can be looked at with less emotional energy, in a more objective manner. When we get to that point, we can make decisions about how to act on them. At this stage, we have choices and our actions are not ruled by the "unclaimed" emotion. For example, a person dealing with shock and disbelief will find it difficult to make quick, sometimes important decisions. If this person is able to name their shock and disbelief, and to accept that this is how they are feeling at this time, they are more able to ask what their options are, or to ask another person to deal with certain decisions they find difficult at this time, or to ask how long they might have before a decision needs to be made, or to get some rest so that they are more alert the next day. Without recognizing their feelings they might push forward, making decisions that are not in the best interest of the patient.

Whatever your experience of dealing with your feelings, during this difficult and stressful time you need to put aside any messages you may have had about the "rightness" or "wrongness" of feelings and begin to make them your friends. In learning to name, claim and tame your own feelings you will become a better listener and helper for your loved one who will need to explore and deal with many feelings in the days and years to come. Further, you will assist yourself in befriending your own experience and learning from it.

Abba God, I feel so much I can hardly express it. There are so many feelings swirling around within me. I don't always know how to respond to what I feel. Sometimes I don't express my feelings well. Help me, O God, to understand what is happening within me and give me the strength to embrace my feelings so that they can become friends to me and not enemies. Amen.

Using the list of feeling words below, or others, choose those that you have felt during a traumatic experience and write about the circumstances surrounding each feeling. What goal or self-esteem issue was involved?

fear	depression	comfort
anger	peace	safety
shock	frustration	support
sadness	confusion	hope
hostility	anxiety	despair
numbness	insecurity	

Chapter Four

Assert Yourself with Medical Personnel

In every profession there are people who have the skills of the profession but not the heart. They know how to perform the tasks; but they haven't mastered the art of dealing with people. The medical profession is no exception. Education or longevity in a profession does not guarantee a compassionate and sensitive practitioner. It is up to patients and their families to teach medical personnel what patients need and how to offer it. It's not what they say, it's how they say it. Do yourself, your loved one and the world a favor: don't put up with "attitude" from doctors, nurses or technicians who treat your loved one or deal with you. Instead, teach them what they need to know. If they don't learn; don't allow them to serve you. If you find medical personnel who treat you and your loved one with respect, attentive listening and compassion, tell them why you think they are great.

THE morning after Joe's surgery, at about 6:30 a.m., I stumbled into the neurological intensive care unit to check on Joe. I'd had three hours of rest and didn't stop to wash or freshen up. I just wanted to see him. As I entered the unit, doctors, in groups because this was a teaching hospital, were making rounds. A group was walking out of Joe's room when I turned the corner. I recognized the surgeon who had reassured me that my husband had an excellent chance of recovery based on the way he had survived the surgery.

As the group approached, an older doctor I had never seen, stepped forward. As the nurse introduced us, he said, "Your husband has survived the surgery. He has a fifty-fifty chance to live through the next few days and come out of his coma. If he does, he has a fifty-fifty chance to live a somewhat normal life. Nothing is for sure and you should be prepared for none of this happening. Do you have any questions?"

I was shocked. I wanted to say, "Does your mother know you talk to people this way? Is she horrified? Who do you think you are? Didn't anyone ever teach you to say hello before you drop a bomb? Will I have to pay you to be treated in this manner?" Instead of speaking these thoughts I looked directly at our surgeon, who was looking at the floor, and asked, "What happened to the good news of yesterday and the reassuring hope for a positive outcome? Don't you doctors ever talk to one another and get your speeches straight?" With this, I walked to the waiting room, sat down and burst into tears. The nurse followed me and as she comforted me, said, "You know, some of the most talented surgeons don't have a clue how to deal with people. He's one of them. Maybe the next family he meets today will be treated a little better."

Both of those encounters have something to teach us:

1. Doctors (or any medical personnel) are human; not gods. As humans they can make mistakes. As humans they can be told when they do. Don't allow arrogance or rudeness or insensitivity to go unchallenged, especially when you are paying for their service.
2. Doctors, in particular, need to be reminded that theirs is a service profession, regardless of the lucrative living it provides. In a service profession, the client has options and the client deserves respect. Don't allow yourself to be disrespected by anyone, especially those whose job it is to serve you. If you don't feel respected, fire the servants and get new ones.
3. There are medical personnel who are sensitive to the feelings and needs of family members and who go out of their way to do whatever they can to assist.
4. When you stand up for yourself and/or your loved one, you might just be helping others, as well.

Questions you should feel free to ask until you receive a clear and satisfactory response:

1. Will my loved one live?
2. What are the consequences of this decision you are asking me to make? Will it allow my loved one a better life? Is there an alternative or less invasive procedure or medicine that will afford a similar or better long-term result?

3. How many of these procedures have you performed? What percentage of these have been successful?
4. Is this procedure/medicine/equipment medically necessary to save or treat my loved one? Is this procedure/medicine/equipment covered by my insurance?
5. How long do I have before I need to make this decision? What will happen if I miss the deadline?
6. Is there someone you would recommend for a second opinion?
7. What are the side-effects of this medicine/procedure? Is there another medicine or procedure you can prescribe with less serious side-effects?

God of all those who suffer, bless our doctors, nurses, technicians and aides. Give them loving and compassionate hearts. Fill them with a passion not only to make the body well; but also, to touch and heal the soul of both patients and their families. Create bonds of openness, listening and respect among all those who care for my loved one. Amen.

Stop and describe the medical personnel with whom you have been dealing.

- Are there some who have gone the extra mile?
- Are there those with whom you are not comfortable? Why?

- Is there something that needs to be said or done in relation to any of these people?
- Do you need to say thanks or bring in some flowers for caring and sensitive caregivers?
- Do you need to ask for a conference to discuss your feelings or to get more information?
- Do you know if there is a chaplain or a patient advocate who could help you?

Chapter Five

The Patient and Family Bill of Rights

If you don't know your rights or the patient's bill of rights, you cannot assure that they will be respected. At this time there is no universal federal Bill of Rights for patients. However, every medical facility has a patient bill of rights, as do most states. Do a little homework and find out what your loved one's rights are.

MOST people approach hospitals, clinics and medical personnel with an attitude of surrender. We raise the white flag because the health care system's way of providing medical assistance is so complex, sterile and intimidating we would rather surrender to it than summon the energy needed to make it work in the optimum way.

As caregivers, we are already expending so much energy just to survive, that dealing with language we don't understand, personnel who would rather not have us "in the way," and rules and policies that were not written with families in mind, is often more than we feel we can bear.

Take heart. While this is a true scenario, there are also some very basic rights that no one should surrender.

Every state, licensed medical facility and clinic has a patient's bill of rights. The Bill of Rights developed by the American Hospital Association in 1976 and revised in 1992 is a model followed by most others. Familiarize yourself with this model and then obtain a copy of the Bill of Rights in the state where your loved one is receiving care and/or in your home state. Compare the two.

With the realization that you actually have rights, comes more confidence in requesting information, being involved in care decisions, working out financial payment arrangements and a whole range of other issues with which you will surely deal.

As you move from institution to institution and facility to facility, don't forget to ask for the Bill of Rights. The very fact that you ask will alert personnel to your attentiveness and to your intention of being a partner in this healing process.

Reflecting on Patient Rights

The American Hospital Association Bill of Rights lists twelve rights that patients should be able to expect. If the patient is not able to exercise these rights on their own behalf because of age, mental ability or severity of illness, then their proxy decision-maker or legally designated medical surrogate may do so. As one of these people, you have the right to be sure your loved one's rights are protected.

A bill of rights generally covers four categories. This next section will review these categories briefly. For more detailed information, research your medical facilities' bill of rights and that of the American Hospital Association.

Patients have a right to:

1. Respect

Every human being has dignity by reason of the fact that they exist. Every human being is created in the image of God, the creator, and because of this is worthy of respect—whether or not their socioeconomic, psychic or physical person is attractive or sympathetic.

Those who are ill have the right to be treated with consideration and respect for their bodily integrity and modesty, their pain management, their time and their value as a person.

Further, respect extends to how the patient is involved in medical decisions, whether or not their religious preferences are acknowledged and appropriately addressed, whether or not proposed medical actions are ethical and humane. Because many people do not understand the language or procedures of the medical world, especially when they are ill and anxious, it would be easy for them to be by-passed in decision-making and/or persuaded to make decisions which are not in line with their own religious and moral beliefs. In an age where research studies and experimentation abound, patients and their families are wise to investigate thoroughly before agreeing to procedures or medications. The more the patient and or his/her caregiver is engaged in the process, the more the patient's rights will be upheld.

Finally, respect extends, as well, to how the patient is treated when conflicts or disagreements arise. Every patient has a right to due process, to be represented in a dispute by an objective decision-maker. Just as a patient should be able to know and understand treatment suggestions before deciding on them, patients should also know the costs of such treatments, who else might be affected by their decisions and whether or not the facility/personnel will work with them to devise responsible and reasonable payment plans.

All of these areas flow seamlessly when respect is present. In most cases, patients and their families don't need to think about many of these issues because facilities and medical personnel have incorporated respect into their overall philosophy, mission and behavior. However, when it is absent, it is usually glaring and a patient has a right to expect better.

2. Accurate and timely information

Patients have a right to know and understand any and all relevant information related to their illness and treatment. Most facilities and doctors will encourage full disclosure of information and will assist the patient in obtaining it. However, some patients don't realize that a few sentences of dialogue are not enough to make good medical decisions. Of course, refusal on the part of a facility or doctor to give accurate information violates patient rights. And the right to timely information includes the present and long-term financial ramifications of medical decisions.

At times, especially during emergencies or when a patient is mentally incapacitated, physicians may need to make decisions without getting the patient's consent and without time to fully discuss specific treatments, risks, consequences, alternatives and the like. But these occasions are the exception, not the norm.

In the case of traumatic injuries, the initial medical decisions may have been made at an accident scene or when a patient was alone and unable to communicate. Sometimes these initial decisions, while appropriate to the moment of emergency, cause more difficult decisions "down the road." Life isn't black and white. Not every decision turns out with a happy ending. However, as soon as possible after the patient regains consciousness or the authorized caregiver arrives, the patient's right to a full disclosure of information and alternatives should be engaged.

3. Privacy and confidentiality

It may seem obvious, but patients have a right to privacy. No patient should learn that their illness, financial or personal information is known or discussed by anyone other than the patient and those who "need to know" in order to offer excellent care. A patient should expect to discuss his/her case in a place not open to the public. They should expect to be examined in privacy with only those needed in attendance. They should be able to receive treatment away from the scrutiny or observation of those not involved in their treatment. They have a right to ask for this without fear of less excellent care.

Privacy also covers a patient's medical records and communication with medical personnel. This is confidential information and the patient has a right to determine who has access to that information. Of course there are exceptions if there is any suspicion of abuse or public health hazard; but under normal circumstances, confidentiality of patient information is legally binding. That's one reason it is important to read and understand everything you are signing, especially if it pertains to who may have access to your personal or medical information. A patient also has the right to review all of this information for accuracy and to file a complaint or ask for changes if they disagree with what they find.

Privacy includes your right to know who is treating you and what their role is in your care. Especially in teaching hospitals or other facilities, there can be many people in and out of a patient's room or treatment area in the course of a day. A patient (or caregiver) is entitled to see the identity of each person who comes into the room, offers treatment or asks for information. They should have their badges clearly visible and be able to explain why they are authorized to deal with this patient. Certainly, patients should be careful of sharing information or allowing any procedures by anyone who may indicate they are a volunteer. If there is any doubt or "intuitive" anxiety about someone who enters a patient's room, the patient or caregiver should feel free to contact the nurses' station and or to refuse information or to cooperate with a procedure until the doubt is clarified.

The right to privacy and confidentiality is a manifestation of respect. Expect both.

4. Control over medical decisions

Every patient has a right to make decisions about their own care before the care is given and during each phase of treatment. Patients may refuse certain types of care or treatment based on the law, hospital policy and religious beliefs. Patients have a right to understand the consequences of all decisions before they make them.

One of the areas that is sometimes difficult in our age of advanced medicine is the role of the "advance directive" such as a living will, health care proxy or durable power of attorney for health care. Not everyone has made these provisions and even when they exist we sometimes hear that they are not followed as the patient intended. Especially in the case of traumatic injuries, even the best organized and most carefully prepared directives may not be helpful if an emergency occurs where there is no one who is aware of their existence. In the best case scenario, patients will be able to inform the doctors and admitting personnel of the existence of their documents and what they wish in case they are unable to make their wishes known in an emergency. Patients have a right to expect that their wishes are honored.

Responsibilities of the Patient and Caregiver

The best medical care occurs when patients and their families are active participants in the health care plan. This implies that not only do patients have rights but they have responsibilities as well.

Just as a patient has the right to expect accurate and timely information, they have a responsibility to provide information about past illnesses, medications, financial or health insurance indicators, and other matters related to or affecting their health status.

Patients have a responsibility to research their illness, to request second opinions and to do their best to obtain as much information as necessary to clarify their health status or to make responsible decisions about treatment.

Just as patients should expect their physicians and institutions to honor their treatment wishes, they have a responsibility to be sure that they have advance directives in place and that a copy of this is accessible to their caregivers.

Further, patients need to be honest about their willingness and/or ability to follow the prescribed health care plan. It will do no one any good and could cause harm if a patient is discharged with a treatment plan that they refuse to follow or which they are unable to follow. By offering honest feedback, often alternative plans can be arranged that will be more beneficial to the patient. Physicians and health care facilities are not mind-readers. Good health care depends on honest interaction and disclosure.

Finally, patients have a responsibility to understand their place in the activity of busy health care institutions that are trying to treat many people. While every patient has a right to effective and timely treatment, sometimes patients have to wait while those with more urgent needs are treated. Making reasonable accommodation to the needs of the hospital and staff is expected, just as offering accurate information and agreeing to an acceptable financial plan.

The more a patient becomes part of the team and takes responsibility for his or her health both prior to and while receiving health care, the happier everyone will be and the better chance there is that everyone's rights will be honored.

God who has given us life, show yourself. Because we are made in your image and likeness we deserve to give and to receive respect. We deserve kindness and assistance as brothers and sisters in your sight. These days are very difficult. I want to be the best partner I can be with the healing team and with my loved one. Help me to understand my loved one's rights so that I can facilitate dialogue and communication, ask the right questions, understand when there is a problem and have the courage to speak up. Be with me as I learn to be an advocate for another. Surround me with your strength and your truth. Enfold me in the protective wings of your angels. Give me a peaceful heart, a discerning eye and compassionate words. Stand with me as I stand with the one I love. Amen.

Take some time to research the Patient's Bill of Rights of the health care facility your loved one is now in or dealing with. Go online to research the Bill of Rights in your state.

Chapter Six

Learn All You Can: Knowledge Is Power

Keep in mind that there is life for the caregiver after the traumatic injury or illness of a loved one. While it will be different, sometimes extremely different, it is still life. No two injuries are alike because different areas of the brain and body are affected with each injury and the effects are multiple. Brain injuries are different from other types of traumatic injuries and even from each other. All traumatic injuries have some things in common. Don't be intimidated by words you don't understand or explanations that seem too complex. Feel free to ask the speaker to explain it in terms you can understand and ask all the questions you want until you have the information you need. If you feel inclined, spend some time in the medical library of the hospital reading about the injury your loved one has so that you can better participate in medical discussions and decisions.

ONE of the most helpful and positive things I did immediately after Joe's brain injury was to spend many hours in the hospital's medical library reading everything I could about his injury. I learned about the brain and its pivotal role in quality of life. I digested volumes about the implications and possible consequences of injuring the brain, the extent to which medical science could help, and what patients could expect. As a teacher, it was natural for me to want to learn about the situation with which I was dealing. I thought everyone in my situation would do that. Little did I know most people didn't even know the medical library existed. One of the best things caregivers can do for themselves, and ultimately for their loved one, is to learn about the illness they are trying to overcome.

This chapter will not attempt to compete with medical texts or organizations with extensive resources dedicated to individual types of injury. Rather I'll try to offer some basic information that will help you to cope with the new world you are entering and some references that will aid in your own research and attempts to prepare an action plan to help your love one.

What is a traumatic injury?

A traumatic injury involves significant tissue, soft-tissue, muscle or structural injury as a result of impact or collision associated with large forces.

Traumatic injuries often occur as a result of transportation accidents, self-imposed wounds/suicide attempts, athletic participation, or physical assaults.

They can include injuries such as:

- Whiplash
- Bone fractures
- Articular cartilage damage from joint or disc injury

- Bladder and urethra punctures
- Head and neck traumas
- Muscle strains, tearing and contusions
- TBI/Brain injuries (both open and closed)
- Spinal cord injuries

Whenever bone, muscle or tissue is suddenly and seriously injured it is considered traumatic.

Traumatic injuries may also increase the risk for other psychosomatic disorders such as depression, phobias, panic disorders and substance abuse. Often those who have suffered a traumatic injury will also suffer posttraumatic stress disorder.

Signs and Symptoms to Be Aware of in an Injured Loved One

General emotional responses to traumatic injury include those similar to the ones caregivers experience. The injured may feel anxiety, anger, shock, mood and behavior changes, altered appetite and weight fluctuation, loss of libido, insomnia, depression, and despair.

They may struggle with psychological scars—invisible injuries—such as dreams and nightmares, posttraumatic stress, loss of control/helplessness, loss of power/indecision, and inability to cope with everyday situations or with their particular situation.

Finally, patients may struggle spiritually, unable to pray or fighting doubt in God's care and presence. While many patients express a deeper spiritual life in the midst of their recovery, it is normal for prayer and faith to be adversely affected by the other emotional and physical issues that may affect a person. Caregivers can help in this regard by not expecting certain responses and by continuing to offer positive support, prayer and encouragement.

Terms and professionals you may meet along the way:

- Rehabilitation: the process of rebuilding and regaining functions that are damaged. There is both formal and informal rehabilitation. Formal rehabilitation takes place in facilities where there is a coordinated program provided by licensed professionals. Informal rehabilitation lasts as long as needed and takes place in the home and in the community.
- Audiologist: one who evaluates hearing deficits and aids in the rehabilitation of those who have such deficits.
- Chaplain: assists patients, families and staff to uncover spiritual issues and facilitate spirituality as a resource for recovery. They help patients and families to own and voice their concerns and fears, to pray, to offer consolation. They act as a liaison with medical personnel and the patient's faith community. Chaplains work out of a Pastoral Care department or on referral from local faith communities.
- Clinical Psychologist: one who evaluates and treats emotional problems and works with the injured, couples, families and groups to aid with stress management.

- Neurologist: a physician who specializes in the nervous system and its disorders.
- Neuropsychologist: a clinical psychologist who deals with the cognitive (thought) and personality processes related to brain functioning. A specialist who evaluates through testing, the mental procedures and functions of the brain and plans training programs to bring it back to optimal functioning as quickly as possible.
- Neurosurgeon: a specially trained physician who cares for all varieties of brain problems and performs brain surgery as needed. He coordinates the medical treatment of the patient and decides whether or not there is need for surgery.
- Occupational Therapist: assists with the recovery of functions of the upper extremities to help people gain maximum independence with activities of daily living.
- Physiatrist: a physician who evaluates the impact of TBI on the functioning of the patient's body and assists in overcoming any disability that has occurred.
- Physical Therapist: helps to regain maximum body movement or to prevent further deterioration in an unconscious or non-mobile patient.
- Psychiatrist: a medical doctor who specializes in the diagnosis and treatment of emotional difficulties. They are the only mental health professionals who can prescribe medication.

- Recreational Therapist: specializes in activities appropriate for leisure time and fitness.
- Rehabilitation/Vocational Counselor: a specialist in social and vocational issues who works to develop the skills and aptitudes necessary for a client to return to work and to the community.
- Rehabilitation Nurse: specially trained to care for the patient depending on the stage of treatment. They provide and coordinate all patient care, serve as a liaison to other team members and are often patient advocates.
- Respiratory Therapist: helps patients to breathe adequately as a means of preventing further complications and/or infections; also responsible for maintaining equipment.
- Social Worker/Case Manager: serves as a liaison between the professional team and all other parties concerned with the patient including the family, funding sources, friends, and past or future placements.
- Speech Pathologist/Therapist: helps patients return to normal or alternative patterns of communication and deals with any swallowing problem the patient may have.

Eight things families need to remember when dealing with any traumatic injury:

1. Reinforce the behaviors you would like to see increase and discourage behaviors that may be harmful or are retarding recovery.

2. When safety is not an issue, ignore moods or behaviors that are not positive.
3. Encourage and facilitate talking about the facts of the injury. Ask questions like: "Tell me what happened." "What do you feel when you think about this experience?" "Are you anxious? Tell me about it." "Did you panic when this happened? What did you do?" "Did you think you would die? How did that feel?" "What is the most difficult part of this situation for you?" "How can I best help you?"
4. Model coping styles you would like to see the injured one use.
5. Avoid situations that provoke behaviors you are trying to reduce.
6. Structure the environment; use cues for positive behaviors. Plan rest periods.
7. Redirect the person rather than challenging them.
8. Seek professional help sooner rather than later

If you are going to be an active participant in your loved one's recovery, you need to understand the nature, boundaries and realities of the injury sustained. You don't have to be an expert but to the degree that you understand what is being talked about and what is requested of both your loved one and you, you will be less stressed, less anxious about the wisdom of your choices and more secure in the care you are giving.

One of the more helpful things I did was to contact the Florida State Chapter of the Brain Injury Association of America. They were very gracious in answering questions and sent me a plethora of educational materials. At the end of the chapter I've listed a few organizations that you might wish to contact when you have time. Each has valuable information they are happy to share and you may even find an emotional support system as the days and weeks progress.

Brain Injury Association of America. biausa.org 703-761-0750

Brain Injury Society. bisociety.org 718-645-4401

People Rebuilding and Living In Dignity [PRALID]. brain injury and other neurological disabilities, pralid.org 585-442-6420

Pilot International. pilotinternational.org 478-743-7403

National Resource Center for Traumatic Brain Injury. braininjuryinstitute.com

National Spinal Cord Injury Association. spinalcord.org

National Spinal Cord Injury Association Resource Center. makoa.org

Victim Assistance Association. beta.bja.ncjrs.org

Domestic Violence Association. abanet.org

O Lord, there is so much to learn. It isn't easy to understand the medical language surrounding my loved one's diagnosis and care plan. Sometimes I feel stumped and worried that my decisions won't be the

best. Watch over each and every decision we make. Give our doctors compassion and wisdom. Give our family trust that is tempered by understanding. Give my loved one hope in the power of science and most especially, in the power of prayer. Bring me the support I need to persevere in caring. Wrap me in the comfort of your love and the wisdom of your Spirit. Amen.

Chapter Seven

Ten Survival Skills for Caregivers

There will be times during the healing and rehabilitation process when you will wonder if you can survive the stress of taking care of a severely injured or ill person while assuming additional responsibilities for the details of daily living, not to mention care for yourself. Those moments of overwhelming physical, mental and emotional fatigue can drag you down. It can seem that there is no way out of what, at times, appears to be a nightmare. If you are lucky enough to have caring family or friends nearby, who are willing to bear some of the burden, it will alleviate some of the stress. In any case, you need to master some survival skills if you hope to be healthy for yourself and for your loved one.

I CAN still remember the days I didn't want to get out of bed to face another day at the hospital. The stress of resuming my job, juggling the hospital schedules, sitting in a room with someone who didn't communicate and I wasn't even sure knew me, was difficult to bear. While I had some verbal support from family and friends, it didn't go nearly as far as I needed. I was exhausted mentally, physically and emotionally. My spiritual life was reduced to "help" more often than not. At certain points I realized that I was forgetting to pay bills, battling depression and growing irritable. It wasn't evident every day; but gradually, when I had a quiet moment, I realized I could barely think about the future without tears. I was headed for a royal case of burnout when God intervened and led me to understand I did not need to approach the task of recovery alone, nor as intensely as I had been. I believe that insight saved my life and helped me to be a better caregiver "for the long haul."

Signs of burnout:

- Being physically exhausted, constantly fatigued
- Feeling continually depressed from day to day
- Difficulty concentrating and paying attention
- Being "wiped out," immobilized
- Feelings of isolation and withdrawing from friends
- Becoming overwhelmed and feeling like a failure
- Increasing use of alcohol and/or drugs
- Increasing marital, work and family conflicts
- More frequent personal illness, such as colds or flu
- Feeling helpless, like "giving up"
- Over-reacting to simple frustrations
- Having more frequent angry outbursts

Coping mechanisms are a person's active efforts to resolve stress and create solutions to problems. We all need to learn how to cope because we are continually thrown into new situations for which no one has prepared us. Caring for those with traumatic injuries and illnesses is probably the ultimate challenge to our coping skills. Learning to cope means the difference between survival and defeat. In addition to joining a family support group, try to resume a family routine that is as normal as possible and do not neglect other people in your circle of family and friends. Don't quit your job unless it is absolutely necessary. Schedule relaxation and leisure times and do not feel guilty about it.

The following simple survival skills worked for me. Give them a try. I believe they can help you, too. They are interchangeable and not to be followed in any order, but as needed.

Survival Skill #1: Eat sensibly and get enough sleep

The first aspects of your lifestyle to be altered by this crisis situation are your sleeping and eating patterns. People either emotionally over-eat, eat less than can sustain good health, or eat erratically and without good nutrition. Likewise, the stress of long hours at hospital bedsides, worry and riding the emotional roller coaster can create insomnia or overwhelming fatigue. The combination of poor nutrition, irregular eating habits and too little or too much sleep can seriously affect your health. It can drain your energy, cloud your ability to make decisions, and contribute to depression, irritability and physical inertness.

If you are to be a caregiver for the long term, your first survival skill is to eat nutritious food regularly and to sleep at least eight hours a night. Do whatever is necessary to acquire or maintain these skills. Begin with breakfast before going to the hospital or work, stop for lunch away from your desk or the hospital room, eat a well-balanced dinner, sitting at your table at home or in a restaurant. Drink at least eight glasses of water each day to stay hydrated. Try not to overindulge in snacks, sweets or fast food. Not only will they produce extra calories; they are also low in nutritional value. Try to go to bed and get up at the same times each day. Sleep is your ally. Fueling your body and mind properly will give you a foundation for managing the challenges each day brings.

Survival Skill #2: Exercise

While these first few skills may sound similar to a self-improvement program, the reality is that physical health affects your entire well-being and the basics are necessary whether you are battling a weight problem or an emotional/psychological problem.

Exercise doesn't have to be time consuming or elaborate. Try to get at least 30 minutes each day. Many exercise experts note that even short bursts of exercise can be effective. If you can walk in the morning or a few times during the day it will not only keep you limber, but it will relieve stress, allow you some fresh air and sunshine, and assist in your emotional balance. Take a walk around the hospital while the staff is bathing or working with your loved one; or, if the weather is not conducive to walking outside, then at least walk the halls of the hospital. Begin the day with a walk or a workout before you go to the hospital. A brisk walk up and down halls, including up and down the stairs, will help you to stay in shape and to relieve the stress of constantly sitting at the bedside of your loved one. If you are familiar with yoga, stretching exercises, or deep breathing exercises, include them faithfully in your daily routine. These can even be done in the hospital room. They help you to develop inner calm, focus and emotional stability.

Survival Skill #3: Meditate

Meditation is the art of quieting one's inner self, centering, and allowing oneself to reflect. To achieve quality meditation, certain elements need to be present:

Breathing: Being able to do deep, consistent breathing.

Still Posture: Finding a position of stillness that can comfortably be held for 15-60 minutes. Place feet flat on the floor or in a crossed-legged/lotus position with hands open and lying quietly in the lap.

Comfort with silence: Meditation requires a space full of silence. The silence facilitates going inward.

Freedom from Distractions: If possible, the place of meditation should be simple and free of distractions.

There are many forms of meditation, but relying on any one formula or style is not what is important. The most important thing is the desire to quiet one's mind and spirit and to focus one's energy within, using either a mantra (repeated word or short phrase) or a visual image as the focusing tool.

Survival Skill #4: Allow yourself a good cry

Stoics don't make good caregivers because they stack their emotions, one by one, inside where they can breed illness. Remember when we talked about denial in chapter two? Stockpiling your emotions doesn't serve your goal of survival.

Tears are a good release for some and in the beginning that may involve a good cry every day. As time goes on the need to release fear, frustration, anger, depression and the like may decrease and the need to cry as well. The key here is not to deny yourself an expression of emotion because you think others will object, you won't look "strong," or it may upset someone else. These are your feelings and if a few tears will help you to bear them in a less destructive way, then it is appropriate to put yourself first.

Survival Skill #5: Give yourself permission to laugh

Just as some people can feel guilty crying, others feel guilty enjoying life. There is a misbegotten understanding that since a loved one is suffering, no one else can enjoy or appreciate life. This is wrong.

While it is true that it is more difficult to enjoy the sunshine, hear the birds, go out with friends and family, and "have fun" when a loved one is hospitalized and suffering; it is also true that doing so is vital to the caregiver's ability to offer real care and empathy over many days and months.

The world and life as it "was" is certainly different and probably never will be the same again. However, you did get up today. You are breathing. You do have things to do that will keep the external trappings of life sane. One of the greatest tasks is to keep your internal life as normal as possible.

Laughter is a strong medicine. Numerous studies have proven the medicinal effects of laughter and humor. If you don't believe me, just read Norman Cousins' *Anatomy of An Illness*.

Survival Skill #6: Write in a journal

Writing in a journal is not something that comes easily to everyone. However, it is an ancient way to develop insight into self and to find support.

"Journaling" is often recommended by counselors and spiritual directors. This is a private time and what you express will not be graded or analyzed by anyone but you. It is a way to express externally the thoughts, feelings and concerns that are churning around internally. Over time, you begin to see patterns emerge. You might notice that certain experiences always trigger self-doubt or anger. Or you might see that certain people bring out confidence and others make you sad. Journals can show you what you think about yourself and life. As the Buddha has taught, "What you think, you will become."

If journaling does nothing else but give you a place to face your own thoughts, fears, hopes and sorrows, it will have served an important purpose. Usually, attended to faithfully each day or once a week, it offers a place to discharge pent up feelings and to pray. Yes, often in a journal one finds words being offered to God. In times of crisis those words may be requests for help, for comfort, for patience, or answers. At other times, they may be words of gratitude. Many people are uncomfortable praying aloud in the presence of others. Journaling offers a place to hear the words of the soul and to come closer to the Great Healer.

The mechanics of journaling are very simple: Buy a clean notebook (or specially bound journal), have a pen and keep both with you. When you write—which can be whenever a thought/opportunity strikes you or at a set time each day or week—just write whatever comes to mind. Don't censor your thoughts . . . just write them. Keep in mind that this is your journal. Whenever you pick it up read what you have written previously—at least one or two days past. Over time, the significance of your daily life, people, events and your coping style will become clearer and clearer.

I have a short prayer I like to say just before I journal. Perhaps it will help you or, you may want to compose your own.

O God, you know me totally and completely, my thoughts, my feelings, my hopes, my needs. Be with me now as I write. Give me the grace to be totally honest. Make this a time of healing. Amen.

Survival Skill #7: Take time for yourself

I found that taking time for myself was the hardest skill I needed to exercise. Between working, caring for our home and animals, spending the time allowed at the hospital, taking care of bills, laundry, work assignments, etc., it didn't seem that the day could hold any time for me. And besides, "I'm not the important one right now!" seemed to be the major thought that crossed my mind whenever I seriously considered taking a break.

I was so wrong! Taking time for yourself, even 15 minutes each day, to focus totally on yourself, is time that will save your life.

Women seem to have more trouble with this skill than men. Without going into all the social mores that have contributed to this, the reality is that women have traditionally juggled far more than one full-time occupation. Even though social thought has evolved in understanding women's equality, the hard truth is that practice and expectation have not.

The last priority many women pay attention to is the one that gives them time for themselves, their own wants and needs. When a loved one is in crisis, that only compounds the dilemma. I call this a dilemma because caring for another is a good and noble activity. However, caring for another at the expense of caring for oneself may ultimately lead to problems like resentment, illness, accidents at home and at work, severed relationships and more.

It is when you nurture yourself as well as you nurture others that your caregiving can be sustained. How can you do this?

When my husband finally came home, I asked my daughters-in-law to drive him to and from his rehabilitation once each week. It was a small thing but it gave me a long afternoon to catch up with myself. I also found six people from church willing to stay for one-hour-shifts, at my home, so that I could do errands without worry. They often stayed longer if needed. In the evening, after Joe was in bed for the night, I either took a long bath to soak out the tensions of the day, or shut off all the "noise" and quietly read or wrote in my journal. Some nights it was only 30 minutes; other nights I had a few hours. The issue wasn't how much time but that I knew I would have time for me each day. Anticipating "my time" made the stresses of the rest of the day manageable.

Look at your daily schedule. Who can help you? Where can you schedule a few minutes for a walk, lunch with a friend, a long bath, quiet reading, journaling? If you value yourself and your loved one, you will. Keep in mind the great commandment: ". . . you shall love your neighbor as yourself." If you don't love yourself and take care of yourself, you won't be able to love others. It's that simple.

Survival Skill #8: Enlist the help of others

I mentioned in Skill #7 that I enlisted the help of others in order to make some personal time. Perhaps you don't know who to ask. Look over this list. It may give you some ideas:

Children
Parents
Extended family
Neighbors

Church members
Pastors
Hospital Social Workers and Chaplains
Local Support Groups
Friends
Business people with whom you trade
Co-Workers
E-mail Buddies

Remember, help isn't always face-to-face. Sometimes help looks like delivering something or picking up a meal on the way home. Help might be someone who can read to or sit with your loved one. Help might be encouraging words over the phone or on the computer or in a card. Help might be certain skills, like accounting or mechanical or lawn work. Help often comes in the form of prayers, blessings and rituals.

Because of my long-standing position as Director of Lay Ministry Development for the Diocese of Orlando, FL, my employer announced Joe's injury in our diocesan newspaper. We received hundreds of good wishes from around the country. It wasn't physical help but it sure helped psychologically and spiritually. We also had friends bring the Eucharist to our home, and our parish priest came to offer the Anointing of the Sick. Once you indicate that you are open to help and you need help, many people will step forward. I organized, "Joe's Angels," and they were a faithful troupe for many months as we tried to get life back on track. I definitely could not have done it without them.

Stretch your horizons. No matter how isolated you may feel or how much you believe you can do this on your own, you can't and there are others who are willing if they know you need them.

Survival Skill #9: Remember you are human

Human beings are incredibly complex, resilient, capable and precious beings. We are able to create unbelievable works of technology and beauty. We can think abstractly, concretely, logically and profoundly. We have the strength to bear and raise children, perform monumental physical feats and love monogamously, deeply and forever. There is a reason God placed humanity as the steward of all creation. There is a reason we are the most perfect of all creatures: we are made in God's own image and likeness. When you come right down to it, that is a startling concept to understand. We are a quantum leap beyond ordinary mammals or anything else for that matter. Human beings have souls.

When you face a crisis of any sizable proportion, your complex human system goes into action. Your mind works to figure out the problem and find a solution. Your body begins burning the fuel you'll need to survive this physical, mental or emotional assault. Your spirit, your soul, searches for deeper meaning and tries to keep you focused on what is good in life.

Yet, with all of this, the truth is that you are not perfect. You are not all knowing or all wise. You are not able to leap tall buildings with a single bound; you tire under prolonged duress. Search as you may for meaning and believe as you may that God is with you, you doubt. You are human, with all the glory and incompleteness that implies. Knowing this ought to bring you comfort. Realizing that for all your abilities you can be inadequate to the circumstance at hand ought to lessen the pressure you place on yourself to have no needs.

Unfortunately, it doesn't because like most of us, you live in a perpetual state of denial about your mortality, your finiteness and your incompleteness.

You need to give yourself "a break." You need to be gentle with your failings, your lack of faith, your inability to live up to everyone's expectations, your fatigue. You need to admit that there is only one God and you are not the one. This is good news because now you have Someone you can rely on who does not fail; Someone you can lean against for support, comfort and protection who will not disappoint. As glorious as your humanity is, it is limited. That's not a bad thing. It is an invitation to deeper dependence on God.

Take a moment and write a letter to God, sharing what you need at this moment.

Survival Skill #10: Pray

Prayer is a conversation with a dear friend. It is an honest sharing of yourself with one who will not betray your confidence. It is an encounter of mutuality and respect. You speak and you listen. You offer yourself and accept the gift of Another.

Prayer isn't something you do for someone else, even though we do pray for others. Prayer is something you do for yourself. You need to connect with the divine. You need to communicate with God. Your soul will shrivel up and die without it. You pray because you need it. As such, you don't have to worry about form, time or place. You don't have to be self-conscious about what you say or do.

Prayer can take many forms. The best prayer is the prayer you need right now. The prayer that changes things and people is the prayer in which you are open to change.

Prayer can be as simple as a quiet moment where you allow yourself to be in God's presence. No words necessary. It can be as complex as a worship service with hundreds of people, music, ritual and readings where you feel caught up in the presence of God within the community. Prayer can be thoughts, words spoken or written or read. The best prayer reveals who you really are and waits for God to respond. The best prayer is when you want to know who God is and you ask for it to be revealed.

Some religions rely heavily on their sacred texts as the basis for prayer. Others have rituals, sacraments, or devotions that help people find the words they need to express their feelings and hopes. Whatever is your history, it is important to know that there is no one right way to pray. There are no magical words or actions that make prayer happen.

Prayer is between the soul and God. No matter how many people are present or absent, no matter how many words or actions are performed or omitted, prayer is the conversation—the soul talk—that happens between a human being and the Creator of the universe.

When Joe was first brought back from surgery and placed in the Neurosurgical Intensive Care Unit, I came in and placed his rosary around his fingers. He had a great devotion to the rosary and even though he was in a coma, I thought he might recognize the familiar beads. He also was committed to praying the Liturgy of the Hours, which are set readings and prayers used throughout the Catholic church at defined hours of the day and night. So each night before I left, I would stand at his bed and read Night Prayer for that day. I reasoned he could probably hear me and even if it didn't comfort him, it comforted me.

At that point, I was able to pray a lot. Most of the time it was simple prayer or meditation. Sometimes it was devotional prayer like the Hours or the rosary or other prayers I like. It helped me to believe that someone understood my heart and soul even when I didn't.

As time stretched from days to months, I found it more difficult to pray. My fatigue, insecurity about the future and whirlwind schedule usually left me very little energy or time to focus on prayer. The best I did some days was a weak, "God you know what I need, what we need, help us." It may not have been profound but it was real and I believe God heard me.

Even if you think you don't know how or you've forgotten what it's like, you can pray. Now, as never before, you need your connection to Someone who understands thoroughly and will help you to endure and survive.

Pray. Now.

God of hope, help us all to survive these dark days. Send some light into my darkness and show me the way. Send your angels to assist in the form of other people who care and who can help me to accomplish all that needs doing. Help me to find enough time to rest and recreate. Give me the strength to cope with my frustration and guilt whenever I feel overwhelmed. Give me a grateful heart, O Lord, that I might thank you for those I love, and a trusting spirit, that I might place the life of this one I love so much into your caring hands. Grant me peace. Amen.

The checklist below will help you to stay focused on what is important in your self-care. Without being rigid in accomplishing each item, which will only add to your stress, make a commitment to try to honor yourself as fully as possible each day by doing the things on this list. Make copies of it and leave it in places you spend time so that you will be reminded of what is important. Gradually, attending to these self-care items will become a welcome and healthy habit.

Survivor's Self-Care Checklist

Today I:

__ took time to pray

__ allowed someone else to do chores around the house

__ asked someone else for help with a task that seems too difficult for me

__ took time for exercise

__ talked with someone about my feelings

__ ate three balanced meals

__ slept for at least eight hours

__ cried and laughed when those feelings came

__ learned something new that can help me or another

__ asserted myself with medical personnel when it was needed

__ placed myself, my loved one and my family in God's hands

Chapter Eight

Hope: The Underrated Healer

"I was regretting the past and fearing the future. Suddenly God was speaking, 'My name is I am.' I waited and God continued, 'When you live in the past, with its mistakes and regrets, it is hard. I am not there. My name is not I was. When you live in the future, with its problems and fears, it is hard. I am not there. My name is not I will be. When you live in this moment, it is not hard. I am here. My name is I am.' " [Wall plague at the guesthouse kitchen, St. Benedict Monastery, Snowmass, Colorado]

WHILE we were still in Minnesota, perhaps within the first two or three weeks after Joe awoke from his coma when things still looked quite bleak, a package came for me in the mail. When I opened it there was a small plaque on a stand. On the plaque was the word: HOPE. I broke down and cried.

I had been fighting so hard to hold on to hope, not talking about my fears with anyone, wondering if hope existed. Here in my hand was a love message, not only from a friend who understood at a deep level what was happening within me; but also, from God. God had reached out to me through my friend and reminded me that as fragile and fleeting as hope sometimes is, it does exist and I had reason to hope. It was a deeply moving and healing moment.

So often, in the midst of tragedy and stress, you are most overwhelmed by what you anticipate. You get lost in the "what ifs" and lose your way, your hope. You forget that hope is both outside of you and within you. Can you find your way again and immerse yourself in the great virtue of hope? I know it is possible.

In the liturgy, just before communion, we hear this prayer " . . . protect us from all anxiety as we wait in joyful hope for the coming of our Savior, Jesus Christ." Hope is what humanity needs in this 21st century; it's what all people need as they face life and its unending challenges. Hope is what you need in order to do what is now the purpose of your life.

Hope is the virtue of those who believe that the Holy Spirit, sent by the Risen Lord, works in and through history. Jesus' promise "to be with us all days even unto the end of the world" is fulfilled in the presence of the Holy Spirit, whose gift is hope. You don't know how the challenges you face today will change your life or the world, but you know, through the lens of history, that situations that seemed intolerable and unsustainable in years past have come to good that was not imagined. The early followers of Christ faced persecution and martyrdom and were outlawed as an heretical sect, yet now Christianity is the dominant religion in the world. Various wars over the millennia seemed to signal an end of the world, yet even those countries most decimated by destruction now flourish economically and socially. In the same vein, millions of people cope with the traumatic injuries and illnesses of loved ones each hour of the day, worldwide, and live to see their rehabilitation and peace, new medicines and advanced procedures. What is hope if not a belief that life is more than what is in front of our faces each day?

Hope like other virtues, is a habit. It is something that grows in you and becomes part of your being the more you practice it. Hope involves patience, staying with the present but open to the possibilities of the future.

Here are some ways that you can practice hope:

- Place the word before you wherever you spend a significant amount of time.
- Meditate on the various times in the life of Christ where hope was the result of his actions or experiences.
- For each challenge you face, claim a hopeful ending, e.g., when the doctor says there are no further treatments available, hope sees the possibility of another opinion, experimental research, miracles; when the bills are mounting and you feel financially insecure, hope envisions friends and family who are willing to secure a loan or make a donation.
- Instead of meeting life's challenges from a posture of negativity (the glass is half empty, nothing can be done); meet challenges with a positive outlook (the glass is half full, there are always creative options).

- Place your life, troubles, worries and challenges in the hands of God with sincere hope that God will care for you in ways that are best.
- Look at nature. No matter how violent the storm or chaotic the destruction, nature renews itself and life continues to flow.
- Visualize hope as a spark within you, always available to provide the fire, energy, enthusiasm and drive you need.
- Remember that the cross is inevitable in each life; and so is the resurrection.
- Listen to classical or other instrumental music. Allow it to enter your soul and tap the hope that resides there in that divine spark that inhabits you.
- Read the lives of the saints, especially those who suffered or doubted. Examine how they coped and found hope.
- As limited as your time and energy are, find a way to give service to someone else whose needs are even greater.
- Be patient with all that is unresolved and look toward the future as though it had already come.

O God of hope, fill me with hope for the future.

Chapter Nine

Prayers and Rituals

IN these pages you will find a variety of prayers that you can use alone or with others. Most I have written and are inspired by my own experience and what happened as I attempted to express those thoughts and feelings to God. Some were written by others and I found them helpful.

The reality is that if you are caring for someone with traumatic injuries, he or she may not be able to understand or participate in complex or detailed prayer forms. That's okay. You can pray for them and you can pray for yourself. If your loved one is able to appreciate the prayers and to join in them, by all means include them and encourage them to express in their own words what is on their heart and mind. You, too, should feel free to pray in your own words, having that conversation with God that can only come from your own experience.

You can use these prayers in any way that helps you. Know that as you pray, others are praying with and for you.

A Prayer In the Morning

Good Morning God of all creation. Thank you for a night spent in safety and the gift of a new day in your presence. I praise and thank you for the sunlight visible through my window and the shelter over my head. I praise and thank you for the food I will eat today, the people you will send to touch my life, the opportunities I will have to witness to your love. I offer you today, each moment, each thought, each action, each decision. I offer you my joys and my sorrows. Bless me with your comforting presence, your wisdom and your peace. Amen. (© Linda Perrone Rooney, 2004)

A Prayer for Making a Wise Decision

Come Holy Spirit, source of inspiration and wisdom, be with me as I discern the truth of this situation and try to make a wise decision. It isn't easy to sort out all the complex information before me. I want to do what is right for my family and for all those involved. Help me to be true to your guidance and to make a choice that will enhance life for all those it affects. I make this prayer in the spirit of Jesus. Amen. (© Linda Perrone Rooney, 2004)

Serenity Prayer

Lord God, grant me the serenity to accept the things I cannot change; courage to change the things I can; and the wisdom to know the difference. [Anonymous]

Ritual and Prayer for Inner Peace

Ritual: Before this prayer, find a comfortable position. Place your feet on the floor and your hands, open in your lap. Inhale deeply through the nose to the count of five. Exhale slowly through the mouth to the count of five. Continue this process until you experience a state of calm.

Gentle and Loving God, be with me now. My inner spirit is restless and in need of peace. Send your angel of comfort to me. Calm my mind and heart and spirit. Heal the fears, hurts and needs that take away my peace. Forgive my doubt. Pour your Holy Spirit into my heart and renew my drooping spirit. (© Linda Perrone Rooney, 2004)

Ritual and Prayer for One Who is Sick

Dear Jesus, Healer of those who come to you in faith, you went about doing good and assisting those who were in need, especially the sick. Come now and bless, (say the person's name as you make a sign of the cross over him/her). Heal (name) from all physical (trace a sign of the cross on the hands), mental (trace a sign of the cross on the forehead), emotional (trace a sign of the cross over the heart) or spiritual illness. Give strength to the body, courage to the spirit, and patience in endurance. Open your heart of compassion and pour it upon your beloved. Amen. (©Linda Perrone Rooney, 2004)

Psalm 23

The Lord is my shepherd, I shall not be in want.
 He makes me lie down in green pastures
he leads me beside quiet waters,
 he restores my soul.
He guides me in paths of righteousness
 for his name's sake.
Even though I walk
 through the valley of the shadow of death,
I will fear no evil,
 for you are with me;

your rod and staff,
they comfort me.

You prepare a table before me
in the presence of my enemies.
You anoint my head with oil;
my cup overflows.
Surely goodness and love will follow me
all the days of my life,
and I shall dwell in the house of the Lord forever.

Prayer of Solace

May Christ support us all the day long, till the shadows lengthen, and the evening comes, and the busy world is hushed, and the fever of life is over and our work is done. Then in His mercy may He give us a safe lodging, and holy rest and peace at last. Amen. (Attributed to John Cardinal Newman).

A Litany of Hope

[The response after each invocation/phrase is: strengthen our hope*].*

O God of all those who fear the future . . .

Creator God, your hope in humankind released the person of Jesus . . .

Jesus, Son of God, your hope in the Father never faltered . . .

Holy Spirit, Source of hope and inspiration for all hearts . . .

Mary, Mother of Jesus, your hope in God's promises gave flesh to our Savior . . .

St. Peter, you hoped in the forgiveness of Jesus . . .
St. Paul, you hoped that your sins of oppression could be transformed into holiness . . .
St. Mary Magdalene, you hoped that the Rabbi, Jesus, would recognize and bless your great love . . .
SS. Mary and Martha, you hoped that Jesus would raise to life your brother, Lazarus . . .
Mother Teresa, you hoped that your care of the most destitute would create something beautiful for God . . .
Bishop Oscar Romero, you hoped that the Salvadoran people would be saved by Christ's love . . .
Blessed Pope John XXIII, your hope in God's people changed the Church . . .
All those who are sick and hope in God's healing . . .
All those who grieve and hope in new life and peace . . .
All those who want to despair but continue to believe in God's loving presence and help . . .

Let us pray: God of all who struggle, be with me. Send your Spirit of comfort and of hope to open my heart to your presence and your power. Help me to stand strong in the face of adversity. Fire up my hope. Let it burn strong and clear for all to see so that I may praise your name always, and under all circumstances and bring you glory. Amen (© Linda Perrone Rooney, 2004)

A Ritual for Leaving Your Loved One Each Day

When it is time to leave your loved one for the day, create a special time of prayer.

- Sit on the side of the bed or at the bedside
- Take hold of your loved one's hands
- [If they are able to understand your words and participate do the following:
  - Ask: Is there anyone we should pray for today before we rest?
    - Anyone who has been kind and helpful?
    - Anyone who came to visit?
    - Anyone you love but have not seen yet?
  - Say: Let's ask God for a special blessing before we rest . . .
    - What type of blessing do you need?
    - [Speak your own need]
  - Do: Bring your loved one's hands to your lips and kiss them saying
    - "May God protect you while we are apart and give you a time of rest." [If there is a prayer that both of you know and would like to add, do so now, e.g., Our Father].

The Five Hopeful Mysteries of the Rosary[1]

The Catholic devotion known as the rosary is a traditional prayer that dynamically connects one to Jesus who acts in the world, by meditating on the various mysteries of his life.

Traditionally, there are fifteen mysteries. The Joyful Mysteries recall the Incarnation, Visitation, Nativity, Presentation in the Temple, and Finding in the Temple.

The Sorrowful Mysteries remember the Agony in the Garden, Scourging at the Pillar, Crowning with Thorns, Carrying of the Cross, and the Crucifixion. The Glorious Mysteries invoke the Resurrection, Ascension, Descent of the Holy Spirit, Assumption of Mary, and Coronation of Mary as Queen of Heaven.

Like the others, the Hopeful Mysteries proclaim that we are the incarnation of Jesus. We give flesh and blood to his Spirit and keep this hope alive in the world.

How to pray the rosary: [You may use rosary beads to help you "keep count" or simply pray the prayers.]

- It is a prayer of meditation, best prayed slowly
- Each "mystery" is composed of one Our Father, ten Hail Mary's and one Glory Be to the Father.
- Pronounce the mystery you wish to reflect on and then begin with the Our Father. Follow it with ten Hail Mary's and end with the Glory Be.
- As you recite the prayers, try to stay focused on the Scripture story that informs each mystery.

The First Hopeful Mystery: Jesus is Baptized and Goes into the Desert. Jesus discovers the meaning of his experience and clarifies his mission. His temptation in the desert leads to renewed strength and hope. He models for us the way to pass through our own times of challenge, struggle, doubt and pain when we renew our trust in God.

The Second Hopeful Mystery: Jesus Invites His Disciples to Work for the Kingdom. Jesus' excitement about his mission leads him to invite others to join him. He declares that the Kingdom of God is at hand and that entry into the Kingdom brings liberation. It is a call to community and discipleship where we can be supported and challenged as we try to live the Gospel.

The Third Hopeful Mystery: Jesus Shares with the Crowds the Good News of His Father's Love. Jesus wanders the land proclaiming in word and deed how much God loves us. He invites everyone, especially those others reject, to share in that unconditional love.

The Fourth Hopeful Mystery: Jesus Heals the Sick and Raises the Dead. Jesus lives his hope in God by becoming an agent of healing. His healing is in the form of justice, of new life, of physical, emotional and spiritual renewal, of forgiveness and peace.

The Fifth Hopeful Mystery: Jesus Invites His Loved Ones to Share the Final Passover. Suffering is not unknown to Jesus. As he tried to live out the calling given to him by his Father, he began to experience the human realities of loneliness, misunderstanding, rejection, betrayal, physical pain, imprisonment, doubt, and death. Through it all, he did not lose hope. This is a source of strength and hope to us, reassuring us that Jesus understands our suffering.

---

1 Noe, K. Killian, *Finding Our Way Home,* Washington, D.C.: Servant Leadership Press, 2001, p. 9.

Additional Titles Published by Resurrection Press, a Catholic Book Publishing Imprint

A Rachel Rosary *Larry Kupferman*	$4.50
Blessings All Around *Dolores Leckey*	$8.95
Catholic Is Wonderful *Mitch Finley*	$4.95
Discernment *Chris Aridas*	$8.95
Edge of Greatness *Joni Woelfel*	$9.95
Growing through the Stress of Ministry *Muto/van Kaam*	$7.95
Grace Notes *Lorraine Murray*	$9.95
Healing through the Mass *Robert DeGrandis, SSJ*	$9.95
Our Grounds for Hope *Fulton J. Sheen*	$7.95
The Healing Rosary *Mike D.*	$5.95
Healing the Wounds of Emotional Abuse *Nancy deFlon*	$6.95
Healing Your Grief *Ruthann Williams, OP*	$7.95
Heart Peace *Adolfo Quezada*	$9.95
Holy Human *Dick Ryan*	$9.95
Life, Love and Laughter *Jim Vlaun*	$7.95
The Joy of Being an Altar Server *Joseph Champlin*	$5.95
The Joy of Being a Bereavement Minister *Nancy Stout*	$5.95
The Joy of Being a Catechist *Gloria Durka*	$4.95
The Joy of Being a Eucharistic Minister *Mitch Finley*	$5.95
The Joy of Being a Lector *Mitch Finley*	$5.95
The Joy of Being an Usher *Gretchen Hailer, RSHM*	$5.95
The Joy of Marriage Preparation *McDonough/Marinelli*	$5.95
The Joy of Music Ministry *J.M. Talbot*	$6.95
The Joy of Praying the Rosary *James McNamara*	$5.95
The Joy of Teaching *Joanmarie Smith*	$5.95
Lessons for Living from the 23rd Psalm *Victor M. Parachin*	$6.95
Lights in the Darkness *Ave Clark, O.P.*	$8.95
Loving Yourself for God's Sake *Adolfo Quezada*	$5.95
Magnetized by God *Robert E. Lauder*	$8.95
Mercy Flows *Rod Damico*	$9.95
Mother Teresa *Eugene Palumbo, S.D.B.*	$5.95
Mother O'Mine *Harry Paige*	$9.95
Mourning Sickness *Keith Smith*	$8.95
The Power of One *Jim Lisante*	$9.95
Prayers from a Seasoned Heart *Joanne Decker*	$8.95
Praying the Lord's Prayer with Mary *Muto/vanKaam*	$8.95
5-Minute Miracles *Linda Schubert*	$4.95
Sabbath Moments *Adolfo Quezada*	$6.95
Season of New Beginnings *Mitch Finley*	$4.95
Sometimes I Haven't Got a Prayer *Mary Sherry*	$8.95
St. Katharine Drexel *Daniel McSheffery*	$12.95
What He Did for Love *Francis X. Gaeta*	$5.95
Woman Soul *Pat Duffy, OP*	$7.95
You Are My Beloved *Mitch Finley*	$10.95